My Journey with Ulcerative Colitis: From Fear to Understanding

"What is happening to me? I am fit and healthy? Why am I now running to toilets? Why blood and mucus? I must have bowel cancer!!!" These were my first thoughts at the age of 38 when my life began changing in 2012.

My mum always said that she had a bad stomach and joked, "I like cabbage, but it doesn't like me!" Over the years, her diet became increasingly bland, consisting of what I now recognize as her safe foods.

So, here I was, 38 years old, cycling around 150km per week, not overweight, a non-smoker, but enjoying wine and beer at the weekends while watching my diet during the week. Why me?

I couldn't pinpoint when it all started, but I began making frequent trips to the toilet. While going three times a day was normal for me, this was ridiculous! Every meal seemed to send me running. Initially, my wife thought I might have celiac disease, so I switched to a bland diet, which unfortunately made no difference.

As time went on, the trips to the toilet became more frequent—up to 12 times a day. Mucus, blood, and eventually, agonizing cramps followed. "I definitely have bowel cancer! Why me? This is shit!" I lamented.

This pattern continued for months, gradually worsening. I planned my 40-minute journey to work with three toilet stops along the way. I even had a "go bag," packed with clothing and wipes, like a prepper ready for the end of the world.

Despite still cycling, my energy levels plummeted, and I struggled with fatigue. Then came the day when everything changed.

I was in a meeting when I had to excuse myself—running to the toilet, I was met with a terrifying sight: a shocking amount of blood. I cleaned up, returned to the meeting, but the afternoon left me feeling drained. I went home early, only to shiver uncontrollably in bed.

My wife, concerned, called the GP, who, despite my recent visit, seemed baffled. As my condition deteriorated rapidly, an ambulance was called. At the hospital, after a long wait, they considered discharging me. But my wife, always assertive, insisted something was seriously wrong.

Thankfully, they listened. A colonoscopy the next morning revealed an inflamed ulcer in my bowel—finally, an explanation for all my symptoms!

Then came the introduction to enemas—uncomfortable, embarrassing, but strangely effective. After weeks of treatment, I returned home, armed with medication and a newfound understanding of my condition.

But the journey didn't end there. I encountered new challenges, like an anal fistula, which required surgery.

Over the years, there were ups and downs, flare-ups, and setbacks. But gradually, I learned to manage my condition. Small changes, like cutting out milk, made a world of difference.

As of 2024, I'm doing well—no enemas, fewer flare-ups, and a better understanding of what works for me. This book is a reflection of my journey with ulcerative colitis, offering insights and helpful information for others navigating this condition.

Introduction

Welcome to the pages of this book, where the journey of resilience, perseverance, and hope unfolds amidst the challenges of living with ulcerative colitis. As someone intimately familiar with the complexities of this condition, I understand the multitude of emotions that accompany a diagnosis – the confusion, the fear, the uncertainty about what lies ahead.

My own journey with ulcerative colitis began with a seemingly innocuous set of symptoms that gradually escalated into a life-altering diagnosis. Like many others who have received this news, I was thrust into a world of medical jargon, treatment options, and lifestyle adjustments that felt overwhelming and daunting.

Yet, amidst the turmoil, I discovered a profound strength within myself – a resilience that allowed me to confront each obstacle with determination and courage. Along the way, I encountered setbacks and struggles, moments of despair and frustration, but I also found moments of clarity, insight, and profound connection with others who shared this journey.

Through the pages of this book, I invite you to join me as we navigate the ups and downs of life with ulcerative colitis – exploring the physical, emotional, and practical aspects of managing this condition with grace and resilience. Together, we will look into topics ranging from understanding the intricacies of ulcerative colitis to practical strategies for coping with symptoms, finding support, and living a fulfilling life despite the challenges.

Whether you are newly diagnosed, a seasoned warrior in the battle against UC, or someone seeking to understand the experiences of a loved one, my hope is that this book serves as guidance, comfort, and inspiration on your journey towards healing and empowerment.

All the best, Seán

Table of Contents

About the Author

Seán O'Connor is a highly skilled and seasoned professional in the field of coaching and counselling. With many years of experience, Seán has made a significant impact on the lives of numerous individuals, guiding them towards personal growth, emotional well-being, and transformative change.

Seán is the owner of Seán O'Connor Coaching, a coaching practice specializing in empowering individuals to reach their full potential. With a passion for personal and professional development, Seán has been dedicating himself to the field of coaching for the past six years.

Since September 2017, Seán has been actively involved in coaching, partnering with clients in a thought-provoking and creative process. Through this collaborative approach, he inspires individuals to unlock their untapped sources of imagination, productivity, and leadership. Seán firmly believes in the transformative power of coaching and its ability to help individuals maximize their personal and professional capabilities.

In addition to his coaching practice, Seán also conducts training workshops and seminars in various areas. These include resilience and stress management, time management and personal effectiveness, as well as communication and interview skills. Seán's expertise in these areas allows him to provide valuable insights and practical strategies to individuals and organizations seeking to enhance their performance.

With a deep understanding of human resources, Seán also holds a role as a Coach with the HSE, further validating his expertise and credibility in the field. His holistic approach to coaching encompasses a range of areas, enabling him to guide clients through both personal and professional challenges.

Also, as a humanistic-trained counsellor he focuses on the individual's inherent capacity for growth and self-actualization. This approach emphasizes the importance of the therapeutic relationship and utilizes techniques such as empathy, genuineness, and unconditional positive regard to create a safe and supportive space for clients to explore their thoughts, feelings, and experiences.

During his time as a Counsellor at HMP Forest Bank, he navigated the challenging environment of a Category B prison in the UK. In this capacity, he provided counselling sessions to adult offenders grappling with complex needs, encompassing issues related to mental health, addiction, depression, self-harm, and suicidal ideation.

Subsequently, in his role as a Counsellor at Acorn Counselling he undertook similar responsibilities within a small voluntary organization based in Manchester. At Acorn Counselling, he engaged actively with individuals, conducted complex therapeutic assessments, built trust with clients, and provided counselling sessions. His role also encompassed referring clients to healthcare professionals, ongoing monitoring of clients' responses to counselling with meticulous maintenance of clinical records.

His deep understanding of human psychology and emotional dynamics allows him to create a trusting therapeutic alliance, where clients feel heard, validated, and supported throughout their healing journey.

Seán has successfully guided clients through trauma, grief, anxiety, depression, and other mental health challenges, equipping them with tools and coping strategies to regain their well-being and live fulfilling lives.

Seán is known for their warmth, professionalism, and genuine passion for helping others. His ability to create a nurturing and empowering therapeutic environment allows clients to feel supported, validated, and inspired to embark on a transformative journey of self-discovery and growth.

In conclusion, Seán is a highly respected and experienced coach and counsellor, equipped with the wisdom, skills, and compassion to guide individuals towards personal transformation, emotional well-being, and empowered living.

Career background

Seán O'Connor is a highly accomplished health professional with a diverse range of experiences and a strong commitment to making a positive impact in the field of health and well-being. Currently serving as a Project Manager in Arts & Health within the Health Service Executive (HSE), Seán is dedicated to exploring the intersections between creativity and health to enhance the well-being of individuals and staff.

In addition to his role in Arts & Health, Seán holds a significant position as a lay member on tribunal panels for the Mental Health Commission. This involvement allows him to contribute to the fair and just assessment of mental health cases, ensuring that the rights and well-being of individuals are protected.

Seán is also deeply passionate about road safety and has developed the Drive Aware Programme (DAP) as a means to effect positive changes in attitudes and behaviours related to impaired, dangerous, and careless driving. Through his program, Seán aims to promote responsible driving practices and reduce the risks associated with reckless behaviour on the roads. His dedication to enhancing road safety has led him to deliver the Drive Aware Programme throughout the country.

As the founder of Seán O'Connor Coaching, Seán offers personalized one-on-one coaching sessions and conducts training workshops and seminars. Leveraging his extensive knowledge and experience, he empowers individuals to overcome challenges, improve their well-being, and achieve personal and professional growth.

Throughout his career, Seán has held various impactful positions. He served as a Project Manager with the HSE National Clinical Programme for People with Disability, where he played a pivotal role in improving healthcare services and support for individuals with disabilities.

As a Task Force Manager in the HSE Drugs & Alcohol sector, Seán contributed to the development and implementation of strategies to address substance abuse issues within the community.

His previous roles also include serving as the Director of the Dyslexia Association of Ireland, where he championed the rights and needs of individuals with dyslexia, and as the Chairperson and Director of Pieta House, an organization dedicated to preventing suicide and providing support to those in crisis.

Furthermore,

Seán has a unique background in the legal field, having served as a sitting Magistrate/Justice of the Peace within Her Majesty's Court Service. He brings a profound understanding of the criminal justice system and leverages this knowledge to make fair and informed decisions.

Seán 's expertise extends to the field of addiction counselling, having worked as an Addiction Counsellor in both community and prison settings. He has provided vital support and guidance to individuals struggling with addiction, helping them on their journey towards recovery. Seán has also contributed to the provision of counselling services within the prison setting, recognizing the importance of addressing mental health needs in such environments.

Additionally, Seán has made valuable contributions to the criminal justice system as a Drug & Alcohol worker with Probation Services. His work in this capacity focused on assisting individuals in overcoming addiction, reintegrating into society, and reducing reoffending rates.

Media work within TV and radio has provided Seán with a platform to raise awareness about various health and social issues. He has utilized these mediums to educate and inform the public, advocating for positive change and promoting well-being.

Seán 's career began in engineering, where he embarked on a four-year apprenticeship as a fresh-faced sixteen-year-old. He gained invaluable experience working for a large multinational Oil and Gas company, further developing his skills and contributing to the industry.

With an impressive array of experiences spanning healthcare, project management, coaching, counselling, advocacy, and engineering, Seán O'Connor embodies a passionate and dedicated health professional committed to improving the lives of individuals and communities. His multifaceted background and expertise enable him to address complex challenges, inspire positive change, and empower others to reach their full potential.

And for further insights into Sean's career to date please visit LinkedIn

https://www.linkedin.com/in/sean-oconnor/

Here's a quick rundown of Seán's publications to date:

A Therapist's Guide to a Little Bit of Everything: Is a comprehensive and invaluable resource designed to support therapists in navigating a wide range of topics and issues they may encounter in their practice.

From Struggle to Strength: Resilience is a quality deeply ingrained in the human spirit. It is the remarkable ability to withstand adversity, recover from setbacks, and emerge stronger than before. In this book, we embark on a journey to understand the essence of resilience, its significance, and the profound impact it can have on our lives

Feck Off Anxiety: As someone deeply invested in the fields of Coaching and Counselling, I have witnessed firsthand the profound impact that anxiety can have on individuals, families, and communities.

Feck Off Overthinking: Looks into the intricate web of overthinking, seeking not only to comprehend its depths but to provide you, the reader.

Feck Off Depression: This book looks into the complex landscape of depression, unravelling its many facets and providing insights into its various forms, from major depressive disorder and persistent depressive disorder to the cyclical highs and lows of bipolar disorder.

Feck Off Stress: A guide that doesn't just help you cope with stress but empowers you to conquer it.

Embracing Dyslexia: Building Strengths, Overcoming Challenges: The book begins by defining dyslexia as a specific learning difference that affects reading, writing, and information processing, emphasizing that it is not indicative of intelligence but rather a neurological difference in language processing.

Leading in Healthcare Management and Leadership in the UK and Ireland: Exploring the intricacies of healthcare leadership and management, shedding light on effective practices in this ever-evolving field.

Leading with Purpose: A Guide to Being an Effective Chairperson in the Charity Sector of the UK and Ireland - Offering guidance to aspiring and current chairpersons, emphasizing the importance of purpose-driven leadership in the non-profit sector.

Empowering Voices: A Comprehensive Guide to Becoming a Freelance Contributor in Drug and Alcohol Addiction Journalism A resource for aspiring freelance journalists interested in covering the crucial topics of drug and alcohol addiction.

Breaking the Chains: A Comprehensive Guide to Addiction Counselling in Ireland and the UK - Shedding light on effective counselling techniques and strategies to support individuals in overcoming addiction.

Shattering Stigma: This book aims to provide a comprehensive section of mental health services in Ireland, looking into the intricacies of assessment, diagnosis, and treatment.

Drive Aware: "Safer roads for a safer society" - This has been the driving principle behind the ambitious initiative known as the Drive Aware program in Ireland.

Empowering Change: A Project Manager's Perspective on the Disability Sector in Ireland: This comprehensive induction provides you with a strong foundation to navigate your role as a Project Manager in the disability sector.

Balancing Justice: A Magistrate's Journey - Sharing my personal experiences and insights as a magistrate, highlighting the challenges and rewards of serving in the legal system.

Mastering Life Coaching: A Comprehensive Guide for Professional Coaches - Equipping life coaches with the necessary tools and knowledge to empower their clients and facilitate positive change.

Clearing the Air: Smoking Cessation Services in the UK and their Benefits to Society - Advocating for the importance of smoking cessation and exploring the valuable services available to individuals looking to quit smoking.

Engineering Excellence: Unveiling the Potential of the Gas and Petroleum Industry' - An exploration of the gas and petroleum industry, revealing the incredible potential and advancements within this vital sector.

All of the above publications can be found at

https://www.amazon.co.uk/~/e/B0C8G4ZN94

Where you can contact him

Seán O'Connor Coaching

https://www.seanoconnorcoaching.com/

Drive Aware Ireland

https://www.driveaware.ie/

2.   Understanding Ulcerative Colitis: A Primer

Ulcerative colitis (UC) is a chronic inflammatory bowel disease (IBD) characterized by inflammation and ulcers in the lining of the colon and rectum. It is one of the two main forms of IBD, the other being Crohn's disease. While the exact cause of UC remains unknown, it is believed to result from a combination of genetic, environmental, and immune system factors.

Anatomy of Ulcerative Colitis:

1. **Location of Inflammation:** Unlike Crohn's disease, which can affect any part of the digestive tract, UC is limited to the colon and rectum. The inflammation typically begins in the rectum and may extend continuously along the colon in a proximal direction.

2. **Pattern of Inflammation:** In UC, inflammation affects the innermost lining (mucosa) of the colon and rectum, leading to the formation of ulcers, or open sores. These ulcers can bleed and produce pus, leading to symptoms such as rectal bleeding, diarrhoea, and abdominal pain.

Symptoms of Ulcerative Colitis:

1. **Diarrhoea:** The hallmark symptom of UC is frequent, urgent bowel movements accompanied by loose or watery stools. In severe cases, diarrhoea may be bloody.

2. **Rectal Bleeding:** Inflammation and ulceration of the rectum can cause rectal bleeding, often seen as bright red blood in the stool or on toilet paper.

3. **Abdominal Pain and Cramping:** Many individuals with UC experience abdominal discomfort, cramping, and pain, particularly during bowel movements.

4. **Fatigue:** Chronic inflammation and frequent bowel movements can lead to fatigue and a general feeling of tiredness.

5. **Weight Loss:** Loss of appetite, malabsorption of nutrients, and increased metabolism due to inflammation can lead to weight loss in some individuals with UC.

Diagnosis of Ulcerative Colitis:

1. **Medical History and Physical Examination:** Your healthcare provider will review your medical history and perform a physical examination to assess your symptoms and overall health.

2. **Endoscopic Procedures:** To visualize the lining of the colon and rectum, your doctor may perform a colonoscopy or sigmoidoscopy. During these procedures, a flexible tube with a camera is inserted into the colon to examine the mucosal lining and collect tissue samples (biopsies) for analysis.

3. **Imaging Studies:** In some cases, imaging studies such as X-rays, CT scans, or MRI scans may be used to assess the extent of inflammation and rule out other conditions.

Treatment of Ulcerative Colitis:

1. **Medications:** The primary goal of treatment is to induce and maintain remission by reducing inflammation in the colon and rectum. Medications commonly used to treat UC include amino salicylates, corticosteroids, immunomodulators, and biologic therapies.

2. **Lifestyle Modifications:** Making dietary changes, managing stress, getting regular exercise, and quitting smoking (if applicable) can help reduce symptoms and improve overall well-being.

3. **Surgery:** In cases of severe UC that do not respond to medical therapy or complications such as toxic megacolon or colorectal cancer, surgery to remove the colon and rectum (proctocolectomy) may be necessary.

Complications of Ulcerative Colitis:

1. **Colon Cancer:** Individuals with long-standing UC have an increased risk of developing colorectal cancer. Regular surveillance colonoscopies are recommended to detect precancerous changes early.

2. **Toxic Megacolon:** Severe inflammation of the colon can lead to a life-threatening condition called toxic megacolon, characterized by rapid dilation of the colon and systemic toxicity.

3. **Extraintestinal Manifestations:** UC can affect other parts of the body, leading to complications such as arthritis, skin rashes, liver disease, and eye inflammation.

Conclusion:

Ulcerative colitis is a chronic condition that can have a significant impact on quality of life. However, with proper medical management, lifestyle modifications, and support, many individuals with UC are able to achieve remission and live fulfilling lives. By understanding the basics of UC, its symptoms, diagnosis, treatment options, and potential complications, individuals can take an active role in managing their condition and improving their overall health and well-being.

3. The Early Days: Navigating Diagnosis and Treatment Options

The Journey Begins

The journey of living with ulcerative colitis often begins with a series of puzzling symptoms that may initially be dismissed as minor digestive issues. However, as symptoms persist and worsen, seeking medical attention becomes imperative. The early days of navigating a diagnosis of ulcerative colitis can be filled with uncertainty, fear, and a whirlwind of emotions as individuals grapple with understanding their symptoms and finding answers.

Recognizing Symptoms

The symptoms of ulcerative colitis can vary widely from person to person, but common indicators include:

- **Diarrhoea:** Frequent, urgent bowel movements with loose or watery stools.

- **Rectal Bleeding:** Blood in the stool or on toilet paper, often bright red in colour.

- **Abdominal Pain:** Cramping, discomfort, or pain in the abdomen, particularly during bowel movements.

- **Fatigue:** Persistent tiredness and lack of energy.

- **Weight Loss:** Unintended weight loss due to loss of appetite or malabsorption of nutrients.

Recognizing these symptoms and their impact on daily life is the first step toward seeking medical evaluation and diagnosis.

Seeking Medical Evaluation

When experiencing symptoms suggestive of ulcerative colitis, it is crucial to consult a healthcare provider for a thorough evaluation. During the diagnostic process, several steps may be involved:

1. **Medical History:** Your healthcare provider will review your medical history, including any family history of gastrointestinal conditions, autoimmune diseases, or inflammatory disorders.

2. **Physical Examination:** A physical examination may be performed to assess your overall health and to check for signs of abdominal tenderness, bloating, or palpable masses.

3. **Diagnostic Tests:** To confirm a diagnosis of ulcerative colitis and rule out other conditions, various tests may be ordered, including:

4. **Blood Tests:** Blood tests may be conducted to check for signs of inflammation (e.g., elevated C-reactive protein or erythrocyte sedimentation rate), anaemia, and nutritional deficiencies.

5. **Stool Tests:** Stool samples may be analysed for the presence of blood, infection, or inflammation.

6. **Endoscopic Procedures:** Colonoscopy or sigmoidoscopy may be performed to visualize the lining of the colon and rectum, obtain tissue samples (biopsies), and assess the extent and severity of inflammation.

Receiving a Diagnosis

Upon completion of diagnostic tests, receiving a diagnosis of ulcerative colitis can evoke a range of emotions, including relief at finally having answers, fear of the unknown, and uncertainty about the future. It is essential to allow yourself time to process these emotions and to seek support from loved ones, healthcare providers, and support groups.

Exploring Treatment Options

Following a diagnosis of ulcerative colitis, exploring treatment options becomes a critical step in managing the condition and achieving remission. Treatment approaches may vary depending on the severity of symptoms, the extent of inflammation, and individual factors such as age, overall health, and personal preferences. Common treatment options include:

1. **Medications:** Medications such as amino salicylates, corticosteroids, immunomodulators, and biologic therapies may be prescribed to reduce inflammation, control symptoms, and induce and maintain remission.

2. **Dietary Modifications:** Making dietary changes, such as avoiding trigger foods, incorporating fibre-rich foods, staying hydrated, and considering a low-residue or low-FODMAP diet, may help alleviate symptoms and improve overall well-being.

3. **Lifestyle Adjustments:** Managing stress, getting regular exercise, prioritizing sleep, and quitting smoking (if applicable) can play a significant role in reducing symptom severity and promoting overall health.

4. **Surgery:** In cases of severe ulcerative colitis that do not respond to medical therapy or complications such as toxic megacolon or colorectal cancer, surgery to remove the colon and rectum (proctocolectomy) may be recommended.

Establishing a Support Network

Navigating the early days of a diagnosis of ulcerative colitis can be overwhelming, but you do not have to face it alone. Establishing a support network of family members, friends, healthcare providers, and fellow individuals living with UC can provide invaluable emotional support, practical guidance, and shared experiences. Support groups, online forums, and advocacy organizations dedicated to ulcerative colitis can also offer valuable resources and a sense of community.

Conclusion

The early days of navigating a diagnosis of ulcerative colitis are often filled with uncertainty, fear, and a myriad of emotions. However, by recognizing symptoms, seeking timely medical evaluation, exploring treatment options, and establishing a support network, individuals can take proactive steps toward managing their condition and achieving a better quality of life. Remember, you are not alone in this journey, and there is hope for a brighter future ahead.

4.Colonoscopy: A Key Diagnostic and Monitoring Tool in Ulcerative Colitis

Colonoscopy plays a crucial role in the diagnosis, monitoring, and management of ulcerative colitis (UC), a chronic inflammatory bowel disease characterized by inflammation of the colon and rectum. By providing direct visualization of the colonic mucosa, colonoscopy allows healthcare providers to assess disease activity, detect complications, and guide treatment decisions. In this chapter, we'll explore the importance of colonoscopy in UC care, including its diagnostic utility, surveillance role, and impact on treatment strategies.

1. Diagnostic Utility of Colonoscopy in UC

1. **Confirming Diagnosis:** Colonoscopy with biopsy is considered the gold standard for diagnosing UC. During the procedure, the healthcare provider examines the colonic mucosa for characteristic signs of inflammation, such as erythema, ulceration, and loss of vascular pattern. Biopsy samples are obtained from inflamed areas for histological analysis, confirming the presence of UC and ruling out other gastrointestinal conditions.

2. **Assessing Disease Extent and Severity:** Colonoscopy allows for accurate assessment of the extent and severity of UC involvement in the colon and rectum. By visualizing the entire colon, including the terminal ileum, healthcare providers can determine the distribution and severity of inflammation, which informs treatment decisions and prognosis.

2. Surveillance Colonoscopy in UC Management

1. **Monitoring Disease Activity:** Surveillance colonoscopy plays a vital role in monitoring disease activity and assessing treatment response in individuals with UC.

Regular colonoscopy evaluations may be recommended to evaluate mucosal healing, detect disease flares, and adjust treatment strategies accordingly.

2. **Detecting Complications:** Colonoscopy allows for the detection of complications associated with UC, such as colonic strictures, pseudo polyps, dysplasia, and colorectal cancer. Surveillance colonoscopy with targeted biopsies may be performed to detect dysplasia early, reducing the risk of colorectal cancer development in individuals with long-standing UC.

3. Impact on Treatment Strategies

1. **Guiding Treatment Decisions:** Colonoscopy findings, including disease severity, extent, and presence of complications, guide treatment decisions in UC management. Mucosal healing, as assessed by colonoscopy, is a key treatment goal associated with improved long-term outcomes and reduced risk of disease progression.

2. **Optimizing Therapeutic Interventions:** Colonoscopy findings may influence the selection of therapeutic interventions in UC. In cases of active inflammation or mucosal ulceration, intensification of medical therapy with immunomodulators, biologics, or corticosteroids may be warranted. Conversely, in individuals with mucosal healing, treatment de-escalation or maintenance therapy may be considered to minimize side effects and optimize long-term remission.

4. Patient Experience and Considerations

1. **Preparation and Sedation:** The preparation for colonoscopy, including bowel cleansing and dietary restrictions, can be challenging for individuals with UC.

Healthcare providers may tailor bowel preparation regimens to minimize discomfort and optimize bowel cleansing. Sedation or anaesthesia is often administered during colonoscopy to ensure patient comfort and relaxation.

2. **Frequency of Surveillance:** The frequency of surveillance colonoscopy in UC management varies depending on disease severity, extent, duration, and individual risk factors. Healthcare providers may recommend surveillance intervals ranging from every 1 to 3 years for individuals with quiescent disease to more frequent evaluations for those with active inflammation, dysplasia, or high-risk features.

Conclusion

Colonoscopy plays a central role in the diagnosis, monitoring, and management of ulcerative colitis (UC), providing valuable insights into disease activity, extent, severity, and complications. By undergoing regular surveillance colonoscopy and collaborating closely with healthcare providers, individuals with UC can optimize treatment outcomes, achieve mucosal healing, and reduce the risk of disease-related complications, ultimately improving their quality of life and long-term prognosis.

5.Understanding Anal Fistula: Causes, Symptoms, Diagnosis, and Treatment

An anal fistula is a common condition characterized by an abnormal tunnel-like tract that forms between the anal canal or rectum and the skin near the anus. While anal fistulas can cause discomfort and complications, understanding the causes, symptoms, diagnosis, and treatment options can help individuals manage this condition effectively.

1. Causes of Anal Fistula

1. **Anal Abscess:** Anal fistulas often develop as a complication of an anal abscess, which occurs when an infection forms in a small gland within the anal canal. When the abscess ruptures, it may lead to the formation of a fistula tract.

2. **Inflammatory Bowel Disease (IBD):** Conditions such as Crohn's disease and ulcerative colitis are associated with an increased risk of anal fistulas due to chronic inflammation and damage to the intestinal lining.

3. **Infection:** Bacterial infections, sexually transmitted infections (STIs), or tuberculosis can contribute to the development of anal fistulas by causing inflammation and tissue damage in the anal region.

2. Symptoms of Anal Fistula

1. **Persistent Anal Pain:** Individuals with anal fistulas may experience chronic or recurring pain in the anal region, particularly during bowel movements or sitting for extended periods.

2. **Rectal Bleeding:** Bleeding from the anus, typically small amounts of bright red blood, may occur due to irritation or inflammation of the fistula tract.

3. **Drainage of Pus or Fluid:** An anal fistula may cause the drainage of foul-smelling pus or fluid from an opening near the anus, which may soil underwear or cause discomfort.

4. **Skin Irritation and Itching:** The skin around the anal opening may become irritated, inflamed, or itchy due to the presence of drainage or fecal matter.

3. Diagnosis of Anal Fistula

1. **Physical Examination:** A healthcare provider will perform a physical examination of the anal region, including visual inspection and digital rectal examination, to assess for signs of an anal fistula, such as skin changes, tenderness, or discharge.

2. **Imaging Studies:** Imaging tests, such as an ultrasound, magnetic resonance imaging (MRI), or computed tomography (CT) scan, may be ordered to visualize the fistula tract, assess its extent, and identify any associated complications.

3. **Endoscopic Evaluation:** In cases where underlying inflammatory bowel disease (IBD) is suspected, an endoscopic evaluation, such as a colonoscopy or flexible sigmoidoscopy, may be performed to examine the lining of the colon and rectum for signs of inflammation or ulceration.

4. Treatment Options for Anal Fistula

1. **Medical Management:** In mild cases of anal fistula, medical management may include the use of antibiotics to treat underlying infections, analgesics to relieve pain, and sitz baths to promote healing and alleviate symptoms.

2. **Surgical Interventions:**

    Fistulotomy: A fistulotomy is a surgical procedure that involves cutting open the fistula tract to allow drainage and promote healing. It is often recommended for simple, superficial fistulas.

    Seton Placement: In cases of complex or high-risk fistulas, a seton—a piece of surgical thread or material—is placed through the fistula tract to keep it open and allow for gradual drainage and healing.

    Laser Therapy: Laser therapy may be used to close off the internal opening of the fistula and promote healing of the surrounding tissue.

3. **Biologic Therapy:** For individuals with underlying inflammatory bowel disease (IBD) or immune-mediated conditions, biologic medications, such as anti-TNF agents or immunomodulators, may be prescribed to reduce inflammation and prevent fistula recurrence.

Conclusion

Anal fistulas are a challenging condition that can cause discomfort and complications for affected individuals. However, with timely diagnosis and appropriate treatment, most anal fistulas can be effectively managed, and symptoms can be alleviated. By understanding the causes, symptoms, diagnosis, and treatment options for anal fistulas, individuals can work with healthcare providers to develop a personalized treatment plan and achieve optimal outcomes.

6.Coping Strategies: Dealing with Symptoms and Flare-Ups

Living with ulcerative colitis (UC) involves managing a chronic condition characterized by unpredictable symptoms and flare-ups. Coping with the physical discomfort, emotional distress, and practical challenges that accompany UC requires a multifaceted approach that encompasses self-care, medication management, lifestyle adjustments, and a supportive network. In this chapter, we will explore various coping strategies to help individuals navigate the ups and downs of living with UC.

Understanding Symptoms and Flare-Ups

1. **Symptom Recognition:** Familiarize yourself with the common symptoms of ulcerative colitis, including diarrhoea, rectal bleeding, abdominal pain, fatigue, and weight loss. Understanding your unique symptom patterns can help you anticipate flare-ups and take proactive measures.

2. **Tracking Symptoms:** Keep a symptom diary to track the frequency, severity, and duration of your symptoms. Monitoring your symptoms can provide valuable insights into potential triggers and patterns, enabling you to better manage your condition.

3. **Recognizing Flare-Ups:** Learn to recognize the signs of a flare-up, such as increased frequency and urgency of bowel movements, changes in stool consistency, abdominal cramping, and fatigue. Early intervention during flare-ups can help minimize symptom severity and duration.

Medication Management

1. **Adhering to Treatment:** Take your medications as prescribed by your healthcare provider, even when you are feeling well. Consistent adherence to medication regimens is essential for maintaining remission and preventing flare-ups.

2. **Communicating with Your Healthcare Team:** Keep open lines of communication with your healthcare provider regarding your medication regimen, symptom management, and any concerns or side affects you may experience. Adjustments to your treatment plan may be necessary based on your individual response and disease activity.

3. **Exploring Alternative Therapies:** In addition to conventional medications, consider exploring complementary and alternative therapies such as acupuncture, probiotics, herbal supplements, and mind-body techniques (e.g., yoga, meditation) to help alleviate symptoms and enhance overall well-being. However, always consult with your healthcare provider before incorporating new therapies into your treatment plan.

Lifestyle Modifications

1. **Dietary Modifications:** Experiment with dietary modifications to identify trigger foods that may exacerbate your symptoms. Common trigger foods for individuals with UC include spicy foods, high-fibre foods, dairy products, caffeine, and alcohol. Consider working with a registered dietitian to develop a personalized diet plan that meets your nutritional needs while minimizing symptom triggers.

2. **Stress Management:** Practice stress-reduction techniques such as deep breathing, progressive muscle relaxation, mindfulness meditation, and guided imagery to help manage stress and promote relaxation. Engaging in regular exercise, spending time outdoors, pursuing hobbies, and maintaining social connections can also contribute to stress relief and emotional well-being.

3. **Prioritizing Rest and Sleep:** Adequate rest and quality sleep are essential for managing UC symptoms and supporting overall health. Establish a consistent sleep routine, create a comfortable sleep environment, and practice relaxation techniques before bedtime to promote restful sleep.

Building a Support Network

1. **Seeking Support:** Reach out to friends, family members, and fellow individuals living with UC for emotional support, understanding, and encouragement. Participate in support groups, online forums, and community events dedicated to ulcerative colitis to connect with others who share similar experiences and challenges.

2. **Educating Loved Ones:** Educate your loved ones about ulcerative colitis, its symptoms, and its impact on daily life. Foster open communication and empathy within your support network, and enlist their assistance and understanding during times of need.

3. **Professional Support:** Consider seeking professional support from a therapist, counsellor, or psychologist to help cope with the emotional and psychological aspects of living with UC.

Therapy can provide a safe space to express your feelings, explore coping strategies, and develop resilience in the face of chronic illness.

Conclusion

Coping with the symptoms and flare-ups of ulcerative colitis requires a comprehensive approach that addresses physical, emotional, and practical aspects of the condition. By understanding your symptoms, adhering to treatment, making lifestyle modifications, and building a strong support network, you can effectively manage your condition and enhance your quality of life. Remember, living with UC may present challenges, but with resilience, perseverance, and support, you can navigate this journey with strength and courage.

7.Medications and Treatments: What Works and What Doesn't

Finding the right medications and treatments to manage ulcerative colitis (UC) can be a complex and often challenging process. With a wide array of options available, ranging from traditional medications to newer biologic therapies and surgical interventions, it's essential to understand the pros and cons of each approach. In this chapter, we'll explore the various medications and treatments used to treat UC, highlighting what works, what doesn't, and considerations for individualized care.

1. Amino salicylates

What Works: Amino salicylates, such as mesalamine and sulfasalazine, are commonly used as first-line therapy for mild to moderate UC. They work by reducing inflammation in the colon and rectum, helping to induce and maintain remission.

What Doesn't: While amino salicylates can be effective for many individuals with UC, they may not provide sufficient symptom relief for those with more severe disease or extensive inflammation. Additionally, some people may experience side effects such as nausea, diarrhoea, headache, and allergic reactions.

2. Corticosteroids

What Works: Corticosteroids, such as prednisone and budesonide, are potent anti-inflammatory medications used to control moderate to severe UC flare-ups. They are typically prescribed for short-term use to induce remission during acute episodes.

What Doesn't: Long-term use of corticosteroids is associated with significant side effects, including weight gain, mood changes, insomnia, osteoporosis, and increased susceptibility to infections. Therefore, they are not recommended for maintenance therapy or prolonged use in UC.

3. Immunomodulators

What Works: Immunomodulators, such as azathioprine, 6-mercaptopurine, and methotrexate, work by suppressing the immune system to reduce inflammation in UC. They are often used as steroid-sparing agents or in combination with other medications to maintain remission.

What Doesn't: Immunomodulators may take several weeks to months to exert their full therapeutic effect, and some individuals may not respond adequately to these medications. Additionally, they carry risks of side effects, including bone marrow suppression, liver toxicity, pancreatitis, and increased susceptibility to infections.

4. Biologic Therapies

What Works: Biologic therapies, such as anti-tumour necrosis factor (TNF) agents (e.g., infliximab, adalimumab, golimumab), anti-integrin agents (e.g., vedolizumab), and anti-interleukin agents (e.g., Ustekinumab), target specific components of the immune system involved in the inflammatory process. They are highly effective in inducing and maintaining remission in moderate to severe UC, particularly for individuals who have failed conventional therapies.

What Doesn't: While biologic therapies have revolutionized the treatment of UC, they are not without drawbacks. They are administered via injection or infusion, which may be inconvenient for some patients.

Additionally, they carry risks of side effects, including infusion reactions, increased risk of infections, and rare but serious adverse events such as malignancies and autoimmune reactions.

5. Surgery

What Works: For individuals with severe UC that is refractory to medical therapy or complications such as toxic megacolon, perforation, or colorectal cancer, surgical intervention may be necessary. Surgical options for UC include total proctocolectomy with ileal pouch-anal anastomosis (IPAA), ileostomy, and colectomy with end ileostomy.

What Doesn't: Surgery is a major decision that carries risks of complications, including infection, bleeding, bowel obstruction, pouchitis, and pouch failure. It involves permanent alterations to gastrointestinal anatomy and may have implications for fertility, sexual function, and quality of life.

Considerations for Individualized Care

1. **Disease Severity:** The choice of medication or treatment approach should be tailored to the individual's disease severity, extent of inflammation, and treatment goals (e.g., induction versus maintenance of remission).

2. **Response to Previous Therapies:** Consideration should be given to the individual's response to previous medications, including efficacy, tolerability, and adverse effects.

3. **Safety Profile:** Evaluate the safety profile of medications and treatments, weighing the potential benefits against the risks of adverse effects and complications.

4. **Patient Preferences:** Take into account the patient's preferences, lifestyle factors, treatment preferences, and willingness to adhere to therapy when selecting treatment options.

Conclusion

Navigating the landscape of medications and treatments for ulcerative colitis requires a thorough understanding of the available options, their mechanisms of action, and their respective benefits and limitations. By working closely with healthcare providers to develop an individualized treatment plan that takes into account disease severity, treatment goals, safety considerations, and patient preferences, individuals with UC can effectively manage their condition and improve their quality of life.

8.Diet and Nutrition: Finding Balance and Managing Triggers

Diet plays a crucial role in managing ulcerative colitis (UC), as certain foods and dietary habits can either exacerbate symptoms or help alleviate them. Finding the right balance and identifying individual triggers is key to optimizing nutritional intake and promoting gut health. In this chapter, we'll explore various dietary strategies for managing UC, from identifying trigger foods to implementing dietary modifications and maintaining adequate nutrition.

Understanding Trigger Foods

1. **Common Trigger Foods:** Certain foods and beverages are known to exacerbate symptoms in individuals with UC. Common trigger foods include:

   High-fibre foods: Raw fruits, vegetables, nuts, seeds, and whole grains can be difficult to digest and may aggravate symptoms such as diarrhoea and abdominal pain.

   Dairy products: Lactose intolerance is common among individuals with UC, and dairy products may exacerbate symptoms such as bloating, gas, and diarrhoea.

   Spicy foods: Spices and seasonings such as chili peppers, hot sauce, and curry can irritate the gastrointestinal tract and trigger flare-ups in some individuals.

   Caffeine and alcohol: Stimulants such as caffeine and alcohol can stimulate bowel movements and exacerbate diarrhoea in individuals with UC.

2. **Keeping a Food Diary:** Keeping a food diary can help identify trigger foods and patterns of symptom exacerbation. Record your daily food intake, symptoms, and bowel habits to pinpoint potential culprits and make informed dietary modifications.

Implementing Dietary Modifications

1. **Low-Residue Diet:** A low-residue diet limits the consumption of high-fibre foods and promotes the consumption of easily digestible, low-fibre options. This can help reduce stool volume, frequency, and consistency, alleviating symptoms such as diarrhoea and abdominal cramping.

2. **Low-FODMAP Diet:** The low-FODMAP diet restricts fermentable carbohydrates that may contribute to gastrointestinal symptoms such as bloating, gas, and diarrhoea. By eliminating high-FODMAP foods and gradually reintroducing them, individuals can identify specific triggers and tailor their diet accordingly.

3. **Elimination Diets:** Elimination diets involve temporarily removing specific food groups or ingredients from the diet to assess their impact on symptoms. Common elimination diets for UC include gluten-free, dairy-free, and low-histamine diets.

4. **Probiotics and Prebiotics:** Probiotics are beneficial bacteria that can help restore balance to the gut microbiota and improve symptoms in some individuals with UC. Prebiotics, on the other hand, are non-digestible fibres that promote the growth of beneficial bacteria.

Incorporating probiotic-rich foods (e.g., yogurt, kefir, sauerkraut) and prebiotic-rich foods (e.g., bananas, onions, garlic) into the diet may have beneficial effects on gut health.

Maintaining Adequate Nutrition

1. **Nutrient-Dense Foods:** Focus on incorporating nutrient-dense foods into your diet to ensure adequate intake of essential vitamins, minerals, and macronutrients. Examples include lean proteins, fruits, vegetables, whole grains, nuts, seeds, and dairy alternatives.

2. **Supplementation:** In some cases, individuals with UC may require supplementation to address nutrient deficiencies or support overall health. Common supplements for UC include vitamin D, calcium, iron, B vitamins, and omega-3 fatty acids.

3. **Hydration:** Stay hydrated by drinking plenty of fluids throughout the day, particularly water. Avoid beverages that may exacerbate symptoms, such as carbonated drinks, caffeinated beverages, and alcohol.

Working with a Registered Dietitian

1. **Individualized Guidance:** Consider working with a registered dietitian who specializes in gastrointestinal disorders to receive personalized dietary guidance and support. A dietitian can help you identify trigger foods, develop meal plans, optimize nutrition, and navigate dietary challenges associated with UC.

2. **Long-Term Management:** A registered dietitian can assist with long-term dietary management of UC, providing ongoing support and monitoring to ensure optimal nutrition and symptom management.

Conclusion

Managing ulcerative colitis through diet and nutrition involves a combination of identifying trigger foods, implementing dietary modifications, and maintaining adequate nutrition. By understanding individual triggers, making informed dietary choices, and working with healthcare professionals, individuals with UC can optimize their nutritional intake, alleviate symptoms, and improve overall well-being.

9.The Emotional Rollercoaster: Dealing with Anxiety, Depression, and Stress

Living with ulcerative colitis (UC) can be emotionally challenging, as individuals navigate the physical symptoms, lifestyle adjustments, and uncertainty that accompany this chronic condition. Anxiety, depression, and stress are common psychological responses to the challenges of managing UC, but they can also exacerbate symptoms and impact overall well-being. In this chapter, we'll explore strategies for coping with the emotional rollercoaster of living with UC and nurturing mental health resilience.

Understanding the Impact of UC on Mental Health

1. **Psychological Burden:** The unpredictable nature of UC, with its symptoms of abdominal pain, diarrhoea, and fatigue, can take a toll on mental health and quality of life. Individuals may experience feelings of frustration, fear, isolation, and loss of control over their bodies and daily routines.

2. **Stigma and Misunderstanding:** Stigma surrounding gastrointestinal conditions such as UC may contribute to feelings of shame, embarrassment, and reluctance to discuss symptoms openly. Misunderstandings about UC and its impact on daily life may further exacerbate feelings of isolation and alienation.

3. **Biopsychosocial Model:** The biopsychosocial model recognizes the complex interplay between biological, psychological, and social factors in shaping health outcomes. Stress, anxiety, and depression can exacerbate inflammation and symptom severity in UC, highlighting the importance of addressing mental health alongside physical health.

Coping Strategies for Anxiety, Depression, and Stress

1. **Education and Awareness:** Educate yourself about ulcerative colitis, its symptoms, treatments, and management strategies. Understanding your condition can empower you to take an active role in your care and make informed decisions about treatment and lifestyle choices.

2. **Open Communication:** Foster open communication with healthcare providers, loved ones, and support networks about your thoughts, feelings, and experiences. Share your concerns, fears, and needs openly to receive the support and understanding you deserve.

3. **Mindfulness and Relaxation Techniques:** Practice mindfulness meditation, deep breathing exercises, progressive muscle relaxation, and guided imagery to promote relaxation, reduce stress, and cultivate a sense of calm amidst the chaos of living with UC.

4. **Cognitive-Behavioural Therapy (CBT):** Consider seeking therapy with a licensed therapist who specializes in cognitive-behavioural therapy (CBT). CBT can help identify and challenge negative thought patterns, develop coping strategies for managing stress and anxiety, and enhance resilience in the face of adversity.

5. **Physical Activity:** Engage in regular physical activity, such as walking, jogging, yoga, or tai chi, to release endorphins, improve mood, and reduce symptoms of anxiety and depression. Choose activities that you enjoy and can incorporate into your daily routine.

6. **Social Support:** Seek support from friends, family members, support groups, and online communities of individuals living with UC. Connecting with others who share similar experiences can provide validation, empathy, and a sense of belonging.

7. **Self-Care:** Prioritize self-care activities that nurture your physical, emotional, and spiritual well-being. Practice self-compassion, set realistic expectations, establish boundaries, and engage in activities that bring joy and fulfilment.

Seeking Professional Help

1. **Recognizing Warning Signs:** Be vigilant for warning signs of severe anxiety, depression, or suicidal ideation, such as persistent sadness, loss of interest in activities, changes in appetite or sleep patterns, and thoughts of self-harm.

2. **Professional Evaluation:** If you experience persistent or worsening symptoms of anxiety, depression, or stress, seek professional evaluation and treatment from a licensed mental health professional. Therapy, medication, or a combination of both may be recommended to manage symptoms and improve quality of life.

3. **Crisis Intervention:** In the event of a mental health crisis or emergency, reach out to emergency services, crisis hotlines, or mental health professionals for immediate assistance and support. Remember, you are not alone, and help is available.

Conclusion

Navigating the emotional rollercoaster of living with ulcerative colitis requires resilience, self-awareness, and support from healthcare providers, loved ones, and community networks. By acknowledging and addressing the psychological impact of UC, individuals can cultivate mental health resilience, reduce stress and anxiety, and improve overall well-being. Remember, it's okay to seek help, prioritize self-care, and lean on others for support during difficult times.

10.Lifestyle Adjustments: How UC Impacts Daily Life

Ulcerative colitis (UC) is a chronic condition that can significantly impact various aspects of daily life, from physical health and emotional well-being to social interactions and overall quality of life. Managing UC requires making lifestyle adjustments to accommodate symptoms, treatment regimens, and the unpredictability of the condition. In this chapter, we'll explore how UC impacts daily life and strategies for adapting to its challenges.

Physical Impact

1. **Symptoms:** The hallmark symptoms of UC, including diarrhoea, rectal bleeding, abdominal pain, and fatigue, can have a profound impact on daily activities such as work, school, exercise, and leisure pursuits. Individuals may experience frequent and urgent bowel movements, leading to disruptions in daily routines and limitations in mobility.

2. **Medication Side Effects:** The medications used to treat UC, such as corticosteroids, immunomodulators, and biologic therapies, can cause side effects such as weight gain, mood changes, insomnia, and increased susceptibility to infections. Managing medication side effects may require additional lifestyle adjustments and vigilance.

Emotional Impact

1. **Psychological Distress:** Living with a chronic condition like UC can evoke a range of emotions, including anxiety, depression, frustration, and uncertainty about the future. Coping with the physical symptoms, lifestyle limitations, and unpredictability of UC can take a toll on mental health and well-being.

2. **Stigma and Isolation:** Stigma surrounding gastrointestinal conditions and misconceptions about UC may contribute to feelings of shame, embarrassment, and social isolation. Individuals may hesitate to discuss their symptoms openly or seek support from others due to fear of judgment or misunderstanding.

Social Impact

1. **Social Withdrawal:** The unpredictable nature of UC symptoms, combined with concerns about access to restroom facilities and fear of embarrassment, may lead to social withdrawal and avoidance of social activities. Individuals may feel reluctant to participate in social gatherings, travel, or engage in activities outside the home.

2. **Relationship Strain:** Managing UC can place strain on personal relationships, including those with family members, friends, and romantic partners. Communication breakdowns, misunderstandings, and caregiving responsibilities may create tension and conflict within relationships.

Work and School

1. **Work Productivity:** UC symptoms such as fatigue, abdominal pain, and frequent bowel movements can impact work productivity and performance. Individuals may require accommodations such as flexible work hours, telecommuting options, or access to restroom facilities to manage symptoms effectively.

2. **School Attendance:** Children and adolescents with UC may experience disruptions in school attendance, participation, and academic performance due to symptoms such as diarrhoea, abdominal pain, and fatigue. Collaboration with school administrators, teachers, and healthcare providers is essential to support academic success and well-being.

Strategies for Adaptation

1. **Self-Advocacy:** Advocate for your needs and rights as a person living with UC, whether it's requesting workplace accommodations, seeking support from educational institutions, or asserting your boundaries in personal relationships.

2. **Education and Awareness:** Educate yourself and others about UC, its symptoms, treatments, and management strategies. Increasing awareness and understanding can reduce stigma, foster empathy, and promote support within the community.

3. **Self-Care:** Prioritize self-care activities that nurture your physical, emotional, and psychological well-being. Practice stress-reduction techniques, engage in regular exercise, maintain a balanced diet, get adequate sleep, and seek support from healthcare providers, therapists, and support networks.

4. **Open Communication:** Foster open communication with family members, friends, coworkers, and healthcare providers about your experiences, needs, and challenges related to UC. Encourage honest dialogue, active listening, and mutual support within your social and professional networks.

5. **Community Engagement:** Connect with others who share similar experiences and challenges related to UC through support groups, online forums, advocacy organizations, and community events. Building a support network of peers can provide validation, encouragement, and a sense of belonging.

Conclusion

Living with ulcerative colitis requires ongoing adaptation, resilience, and support from healthcare providers, loved ones, and community networks. By acknowledging the physical, emotional, and social impacts of UC on daily life and implementing strategies for adaptation and self-care, individuals can navigate the challenges of living with UC with greater resilience, empowerment, and well-being.

11.Support Systems: Finding Help and Building a Support Network

Living with ulcerative colitis (UC) can be challenging, but you don't have to face it alone. Building a support network of healthcare professionals, loved ones, fellow individuals with UC, and community resources can provide invaluable support, understanding, and encouragement on your journey. In this chapter, we'll explore support systems available in Ireland and the UK, as well as strategies for accessing help and building a strong support network.

Healthcare Professionals

1. **Gastroenterologists:** Gastroenterologists specialize in the diagnosis and management of gastrointestinal conditions such as UC. They play a central role in coordinating your care, prescribing medications, and monitoring your disease activity.

2. **General Practitioners (GPs):** Your GP serves as your primary point of contact for managing day-to-day health concerns, coordinating referrals to specialists, and providing ongoing support and guidance.

3. **Nurses:** Specialist nurses, such as inflammatory bowel disease (IBD) nurses, provide personalized support, education, and monitoring for individuals with UC. They offer practical advice, administer treatments, and facilitate communication between patients and healthcare providers.

Support Groups and Organizations

1. **Crohn's and Colitis Support Groups:** Local support groups for individuals with Crohn's disease and ulcerative colitis offer opportunities to connect with others who share similar experiences, challenges, and concerns. These groups provide emotional support, practical advice, and a sense of community.

2. **Crohn's and Colitis UK:** Crohn's and Colitis UK is a leading charity dedicated to improving the lives of individuals affected by Crohn's disease and ulcerative colitis. They offer a range of support services, including information resources, helplines, online forums, advocacy initiatives, and local support groups.

3. **IBD Ireland:** IBD Ireland is a nonprofit organization dedicated to raising awareness, providing support, and advocating for individuals affected by inflammatory bowel disease (IBD) in Ireland. They offer information resources, support groups, educational events, and peer support programs for individuals with UC and their families.

Online Resources

1. **IBD Passport:** The IBD Passport is an online platform developed by Crohn's and Colitis UK, providing personalized information and resources for individuals with Crohn's disease and ulcerative colitis. It offers practical advice on managing symptoms, accessing healthcare services, and living well with IBD.

2. **Crohn's and Colitis Community:** Crohn's and Colitis UK hosts an online community forum where individuals affected by Crohn's disease and ulcerative colitis can connect, share experiences, ask questions, and offer support to one another in a safe and supportive environment.

Peer Support

1. **Peer Mentoring Programs:** Some organizations, such as Crohn's and Colitis UK, offer peer mentoring programs where individuals with UC can connect with trained volunteers who have firsthand experience living with the condition. Peer mentors provide guidance, empathy, and practical advice based on their own experiences.

2. **Social Media Groups:** Social media platforms such as Facebook, Twitter, and Instagram host numerous groups and pages dedicated to inflammatory bowel disease (IBD) awareness, support, and advocacy. These online communities offer opportunities to connect with others, share stories, and access information and resources.

Family and Friends

1. **Family Support:** Lean on your family members for emotional support, understanding, and practical assistance as you navigate the challenges of living with UC. Open communication, empathy, and mutual support can strengthen familial bonds and foster resilience in the face of adversity.

2. **Friendship Networks:** Cultivate friendships with individuals who offer acceptance, compassion, and nonjudgmental support.

Friends can provide companionship, distraction, and laughter during difficult times, enhancing your overall well-being and quality of life.

Conclusion

Building a support network is essential for individuals living with ulcerative colitis, providing emotional, practical, and social support on their journey. Whether accessing healthcare services, connecting with peer support groups, or relying on the support of family and friends, individuals with UC can find strength, resilience, and empowerment through their support systems. Remember, you are not alone, and help is available to support you every step of the way.

12.Thriving with UC: Tips for Living Your Best Life Despite the Challenges

Living with ulcerative colitis (UC) presents unique challenges, but it's possible to thrive and lead a fulfilling life despite the obstacles. By adopting a proactive mindset, implementing effective self-care strategies, and embracing a holistic approach to well-being, individuals with UC can maximize their quality of life and achieve their goals. In this chapter, we'll explore tips for thriving with UC and living your best life despite the challenges.

1. Embrace Self-Acceptance and Resilience

1. **Practice Self-Compassion:** Be kind to yourself and practice self-compassion, acknowledging your strengths, limitations, and efforts to manage UC. Treat yourself with the same kindness and understanding you would offer to a loved one facing similar challenges.

2. **Cultivate Resilience:** Cultivate resilience by developing coping skills, problem-solving abilities, and adaptive strategies to navigate the ups and downs of living with UC. Embrace setbacks as opportunities for growth, learning, and personal development.

2. Prioritize Physical Well-Being

1. **Follow Treatment Plans:** Adhere to your treatment plan prescribed by healthcare professionals, including medications, dietary recommendations, and lifestyle modifications. Consistent management of UC symptoms is essential for maintaining remission and minimizing flare-ups.

2. **Engage in Regular Exercise:** Incorporate regular exercise into your routine, choosing activities that you enjoy and can safely perform.

Exercise helps improve physical fitness, reduce stress, boost mood, and promote overall well-being.

3. **Prioritize Sleep:** Prioritize quality sleep by establishing a consistent sleep schedule, creating a relaxing bedtime routine, and optimizing your sleep environment. Adequate rest is essential for managing UC symptoms, supporting immune function, and enhancing cognitive function.

3. Nourish Your Body with Nutritious Foods

1. **Eat a Balanced Diet:** Focus on eating a balanced diet rich in fruits, vegetables, lean proteins, whole grains, and healthy fats. Experiment with dietary modifications to identify trigger foods and optimize your nutrition while managing UC symptoms.

2. **Stay Hydrated:** Stay hydrated by drinking plenty of fluids throughout the day, particularly water. Limit consumption of beverages that may exacerbate UC symptoms, such as caffeinated drinks and alcohol.

3. **Consider Nutritional Supplements:** If necessary, consider incorporating nutritional supplements into your diet to address specific nutrient deficiencies or support overall health. Consult with healthcare professionals to determine appropriate supplementation based on your individual needs.

4. Nurture Emotional Well-Being

1. **Practice Stress Reduction:** Incorporate stress-reduction techniques into your daily routine, such as mindfulness meditation, deep breathing exercises, progressive muscle relaxation, and guided imagery.

These practices help promote relaxation, reduce anxiety, and improve mood.

2. **Seek Emotional Support:** Seek emotional support from trusted friends, family members, support groups, and mental health professionals. Sharing your experiences, concerns, and feelings with others can provide validation, empathy, and a sense of connection.

3. **Engage in Activities You Enjoy:** Engage in activities that bring you joy, fulfilment, and a sense of purpose. Whether it's pursuing hobbies, spending time with loved ones, or volunteering in your community, prioritizing activities that nourish your soul is essential for emotional well-being.

5. Cultivate Meaningful Connections and Support Systems

1. **Build a Support Network:** Surround yourself with a supportive network of healthcare professionals, loved ones, fellow individuals with UC, and community resources. Lean on your support network for encouragement, understanding, and practical assistance as needed.

2. **Connect with Others:** Connect with others who share similar experiences and challenges related to UC through support groups, online forums, advocacy organizations, and community events. Building connections and sharing stories can provide validation, inspiration, and empowerment.

6. Set Goals and Pursue Your Passions

1. **Set Realistic Goals:** Set realistic, achievable goals for yourself, taking into account your strengths, limitations, and priorities.

    Break larger goals into smaller, manageable steps, and celebrate your progress along the way.

2. **Pursue Your Passions:** Pursue activities, interests, and passions that bring you joy, fulfilment, and a sense of accomplishment. Whether it's pursuing creative endeavours, exploring new hobbies, or advancing your career, investing time and energy in activities that align with your values enhances your sense of purpose and satisfaction.

Conclusion

Thriving with ulcerative colitis is possible with the right mindset, support systems, and self-care strategies in place. By prioritizing physical and emotional well-being, nurturing meaningful connections, and pursuing your passions, you can live your best life despite the challenges of UC. Remember, you are resilient, capable, and deserving of a fulfilling and rewarding life, regardless of the obstacles you face.

13.Relationships and Intimacy: Navigating Personal Connections with UC

Ulcerative colitis (UC) can have a significant impact on personal relationships and intimacy, presenting unique challenges for individuals and their partners. From communication breakdowns and lifestyle adjustments to managing symptoms and emotional well-being, navigating relationships with UC requires understanding, empathy, and mutual support. In this chapter, we'll explore strategies for maintaining healthy relationships and fostering intimacy while living with UC.

Communication and Understanding

1. **Open Communication:** Foster open, honest communication with your partner about your experiences, needs, and concerns related to UC. Share information about your symptoms, treatment plan, and how UC impacts your daily life to promote understanding and empathy.

2. **Educate Your Partner:** Educate your partner about UC, its symptoms, treatments, and management strategies. Help them understand the physical and emotional challenges you face, as well as how they can support you effectively.

3. **Active Listening:** Practice active listening when discussing UC-related issues with your partner. Listen attentively to their perspective, validate their feelings, and offer empathy and support in return.

Lifestyle Adjustments

1. **Flexibility and Adaptation:** Be flexible and adaptable in making lifestyle adjustments to accommodate UC symptoms and treatment regimens.

Work together with your partner to find solutions and compromises that meet both of your needs and preferences.

2. **Managing Stress Together:** Explore stress-reduction techniques and coping strategies together, such as mindfulness meditation, relaxation exercises, and engaging in enjoyable activities. Supporting each other in managing stress can strengthen your relationship and improve overall well-being.

Intimacy and Sexual Health

1. **Emotional Intimacy:** Focus on fostering emotional intimacy and connection with your partner, even when physical intimacy may be impacted by UC symptoms. Communicate openly about your feelings, desires, and concerns, and prioritize quality time together to nurture your bond.

2. **Sexual Health Conversations:** Have open, non-judgmental conversations about sexual health and intimacy with your partner. Discuss how UC symptoms may affect sexual function, libido, and body image, and explore ways to maintain intimacy and pleasure despite these challenges.

3. **Seeking Professional Help:** If sexual dysfunction or intimacy issues arise due to UC, consider seeking support from healthcare professionals, such as gastroenterologists, urologists, or sex therapists. They can provide guidance, interventions, and resources to address sexual health concerns and improve intimacy in your relationship.

Mutual Support and Empathy

1. **Team Approach:** Approach UC management as a team, with both partners actively involved in decision-making, problem-solving, and support. Collaborate on treatment plans, lifestyle adjustments, and emotional support strategies to navigate UC together effectively.

2. **Offering and Receiving Support:** Be receptive to both offering and receiving support from your partner. Offer empathy, encouragement, and practical assistance when your partner is struggling with UC symptoms, and allow them to reciprocate when you need support.

Seeking External Support

1. **Support Groups:** Consider joining support groups or online communities for individuals with UC and their partners. Connecting with others who share similar experiences can provide validation, empathy, and practical advice for navigating relationships and intimacy with UC.

2. **Couples Counselling:** If relationship challenges persist or become overwhelming, consider seeking couples counselling or therapy with a licensed therapist who specializes in chronic illness and relationships. Counselling can provide a safe space to explore communication patterns, address conflict, and strengthen your relationship bond.

Conclusion

Navigating relationships and intimacy with UC requires patience, understanding, and mutual support from both partners. By fostering open communication, making lifestyle adjustments together, prioritizing emotional intimacy, and seeking external support when needed, couples can navigate the challenges of living with UC while maintaining a strong and fulfilling relationship.

14.Advocacy and Awareness: Making Your Voice Heard in the UC Community

Advocacy and awareness play crucial roles in empowering individuals with ulcerative colitis (UC), raising public understanding, and driving positive change in the healthcare system. By sharing your experiences, advocating for your needs, and participating in advocacy initiatives, you can make a meaningful impact in the UC community and beyond. In this chapter, we'll explore strategies for effective advocacy and raising awareness about UC.

1. Sharing Your Story

1. **Personal Narrative:** Share your personal story of living with UC, including your diagnosis journey, treatment experiences, challenges, and triumphs. Your story can inspire others, raise awareness about UC, and break down stigma surrounding gastrointestinal conditions.

2. **Public Speaking:** Consider sharing your story through public speaking engagements, presentations, and panel discussions at healthcare conferences, community events, and support group meetings. Your firsthand perspective can educate and empower audiences while fostering empathy and understanding.

2. Participating in Advocacy Initiatives

1. **Joining Advocacy Organizations:** Get involved with advocacy organizations dedicated to supporting individuals with UC, such as Crohn's and Colitis UK, Crohn's and Colitis Foundation, and local patient advocacy groups. Participate in advocacy campaigns, events, and initiatives to amplify your voice and advocate for policy changes.

2. **Contacting Elected Officials:** Reach out to your local representatives, members of parliament, and policymakers to advocate for improved access to healthcare services, research funding, and legislative protections for individuals with UC. Write letters, make phone calls, and schedule meetings to share your concerns and advocate for change.

3. Utilizing Social Media and Digital Platforms

1. **Social Media Advocacy:** Use social media platforms to raise awareness about UC, share educational resources, and advocate for policy changes. Utilize hashtags such as #UlcerativeColitis, #IBDawareness, and #UCwarrior to connect with others and amplify your message.

2. **Blogging and Podcasting:** Start a blog or podcast to share your experiences, insights, and advocacy efforts related to UC. Use these platforms to engage with your audience, raise awareness about UC-related issues, and advocate for positive change.

4. Educating the Public

1. **Community Outreach:** Engage in community outreach activities to educate the public about UC and gastrointestinal health. Organize educational workshops, health fairs, and awareness events in collaboration with local healthcare providers, schools, and community organizations.

2. **Media Interviews:** Share your expertise and experiences with UC through media interviews with newspapers, magazines, radio stations, and television programs. Use these opportunities to raise awareness, dispel myths, and promote understanding about UC and its impact on individuals and families.

5. Participating in Research and Clinical Trials

1. **Research Participation:** Consider participating in clinical research studies, patient registries, and surveys related to UC. Your participation contributes valuable data and insights to advancing scientific knowledge, improving treatments, and enhancing care for individuals with UC.

2. **Advocating for Research Funding:** Advocate for increased funding for UC research through government agencies, private foundations, and charitable organizations. Highlight the importance of research in discovering new treatments, understanding disease mechanisms, and improving quality of life for individuals with UC.

6. Supporting Access to Care and Resources

1. **Patient Access Programs:** Advocate for improved access to healthcare services, medications, and support programs for individuals with UC. Support initiatives that reduce barriers to care, increase affordability, and promote equitable access to resources for all patients.

2. **Peer Support Networks:** Support the development and expansion of peer support networks, helplines, and online communities for individuals with UC and their caregivers. These networks provide valuable emotional support, information sharing, and solidarity for those navigating the challenges of living with UC.

Conclusion

Advocacy and awareness are powerful tools for making a positive impact in the UC community, raising public understanding, and driving change in healthcare policies and practices.

By sharing your story, participating in advocacy initiatives, utilizing social media, educating the public, participating in research, and supporting access to care, you can make your voice heard and contribute to a brighter future for individuals living with UC.

15.Looking Ahead: Hope for the Future and Advances in UC Research

As research in ulcerative colitis (UC) continues to advance, there is growing optimism for improved treatments, better outcomes, and a brighter future for individuals living with this chronic condition. From innovative therapies and personalized medicine to breakthroughs in understanding disease mechanisms, the landscape of UC management is evolving rapidly. In this chapter, we'll explore the latest advances in UC research and the promising developments on the horizon.

1. Precision Medicine and Personalized Therapies

1. **Biomarker Identification:** Researchers are exploring biomarkers—biological indicators of disease activity and response to treatment—to personalize UC management. By identifying biomarkers associated with disease severity, treatment response, and prognosis, clinicians can tailor therapies to individual patients for optimal outcomes.

2. **Targeted Therapies:** Advances in understanding the underlying mechanisms of UC have led to the development of targeted therapies that specifically modulate key pathways involved in inflammation and immune dysregulation. Biologic agents, small molecules, and monoclonal antibodies are being investigated as potential targeted treatments for UC, offering improved efficacy and safety profiles compared to traditional therapies.

2. Gut Microbiota and Microbiome Modulation

1. **Microbiome Research:** The gut microbiota—comprising trillions of microorganisms residing in the gastrointestinal tract—plays a crucial role in the pathogenesis of UC. Researchers are studying the composition and function of the gut microbiome in individuals with UC to identify microbial signatures associated with disease activity and response to treatment.

2. **Microbiome Modulation:** Strategies to modulate the gut microbiota, such as probiotics, prebiotics, fecal microbiota transplantation (FMT), and microbial-targeted therapies, hold promise for restoring microbial balance, reducing inflammation, and promoting mucosal healing in UC. Clinical trials are underway to evaluate the efficacy and safety of microbiome-based interventions in UC management.

3. Novel Therapeutic Approaches

1. **Stem Cell Therapy:** Stem cell therapy holds potential for regenerating damaged intestinal tissue, promoting tissue repair, and inducing immunomodulation in UC. Clinical trials exploring the safety and efficacy of stem cell-based interventions, including mesenchymal stem cells and induced pluripotent stem cells, are underway, offering hope for disease-modifying treatments.

2. **Gene Therapy:** Gene therapy approaches, such as gene editing and gene delivery technologies, aim to modify genetic factors implicated in UC pathogenesis. By targeting specific genes associated with inflammation, mucosal integrity, and immune regulation, gene therapy holds promise for precision medicine in UC treatment.

4. Patient-Centered Outcomes Research

1. **Patient-Reported Outcomes:** Patient-centred outcomes research focuses on identifying and prioritizing outcomes that matter most to individuals with UC, such as symptom control, quality of life, and treatment satisfaction. By incorporating patient perspectives into clinical research and drug development, researchers can ensure that interventions align with patient priorities and preferences.

2. **Shared Decision-Making:** Shared decision-making between patients and healthcare providers emphasizes collaborative discussions, informed consent, and mutual agreement on treatment goals and options. By involving patients as active partners in their care, shared decision-making promotes personalized treatment plans and enhances patient satisfaction and adherence.

5. Digital Health and Telemedicine

1. **Telemedicine Platforms:** Telemedicine platforms and digital health technologies offer opportunities for remote monitoring, virtual consultations, and patient education in UC management. By leveraging telemedicine, individuals with UC can access specialized care, receive timely support, and participate in clinical trials from the comfort of their homes.

2. **Mobile Health Apps:** Mobile health apps designed for individuals with UC provide tools for symptom tracking, medication reminders, dietary monitoring, and lifestyle management. These apps empower patients to take an active role in self-management, promote adherence to treatment regimens, and facilitate communication with healthcare providers.

Conclusion

The future of ulcerative colitis management is bright, with ongoing research efforts driving innovations in treatment approaches, biomarker discovery, microbiome modulation, gene therapy, patient-centred care, and digital health solutions. By harnessing the power of precision medicine, personalized therapies, and patient-centred research, we can optimize outcomes, improve quality of life, and ultimately find a cure for UC. As we look ahead with hope and optimism, let us continue to support and advocate for advancements in UC research to transform the lives of individuals living with this chronic condition.

16.Conclusion: Embracing Resilience and Hope in the Journey with Ulcerative Colitis

As we come to the end of this book to living with ulcerative colitis (UC), it's important to reflect on the journey we've embarked upon together. From the initial challenges of diagnosis and treatment decisions to the ongoing management of symptoms, emotions, and relationships, navigating life with UC requires courage, resilience, and hope. In this concluding chapter, we'll revisit key themes, celebrate achievements, and look forward with optimism to the future.

Embracing Resilience

Living with UC is not without its challenges, but throughout this book, you've demonstrated remarkable resilience in the face of adversity. You've faced setbacks with determination, adapted to new realities with grace, and found strength in moments of vulnerability. Your resilience is a testament to your inner strength and unwavering spirit in the journey with UC.

Finding Hope in Progress

While living with UC may present obstacles, it's essential to recognize the progress and advancements that have been made in understanding and managing this complex condition. From innovative treatments and personalized therapies to groundbreaking research and patient advocacy efforts, there is reason to hope for a brighter future for individuals with UC. By embracing a forward-thinking mindset and participating in the collective efforts to improve care and outcomes, we can continue to make strides towards a world where UC no longer holds power over our lives.

Fostering Connection and Support

Throughout this book, we've emphasized the importance of connection and support in the journey with UC. Whether it's leaning on loved ones for emotional support, connecting with fellow individuals with UC for solidarity and understanding, or advocating for policy changes to improve access to care, our collective strength lies in the power of community. By fostering meaningful connections, offering support to one another, and advocating for change, we can create a world where individuals with UC feel seen, heard, and supported on their journey towards wellness.

Looking Forward with Hope

As we conclude this book, let us carry forward the lessons learned, the insights gained, and the bonds forged in the journey with UC. Let us approach each day with optimism, resilience, and hope for the future, knowing that we are not alone in our struggles and that together, we can overcome any obstacle that comes our way. By embracing resilience, finding hope in progress, fostering connection and support, and looking forward with optimism, we can navigate the journey with UC with courage, grace, and strength.

17.Appendices: Resources, Glossary, and Further Reading

1. Resources

1. **Crohn's and Colitis Organizations:**

    - Crohn's and Colitis UK: Website: crohnsandcolitis.org.uk

    - Crohn's and Colitis Foundation (USA): Website: crohnscolitisfoundation.org

    - IBD Ireland: Website: ibdrelief.ie

2. **Online Support Communities:**

    - Crohn's and Colitis Community: Website: community.crohnscolitisfoundation.org

    - Crohn's and Colitis UK Online Community: Website: crohnsandcolitis.org.uk/community

3. **Patient Education Materials:**

    - IBD Passport: Website: ibdpassport.org

    - WebMD Ulcerative Colitis Centre: Website: webmd.com/ibd-crohns-disease/ulcerative-colitis

4. **Clinical Trials Registries:**

    - ClinicalTrials.gov: Website: clinicaltrials.gov

    - European Union Clinical Trials Register: Website: clinicaltrialsregister.eu

2. Glossary

- **Ulcerative Colitis (UC):** A chronic inflammatory bowel disease characterized by inflammation and ulceration of the colon and rectum.

- **Inflammatory Bowel Disease (IBD):** A group of chronic inflammatory conditions affecting the gastrointestinal tract, including Crohn's disease and ulcerative colitis.

- **Colonoscopy:** A diagnostic procedure that allows visualization of the colon and rectum using a flexible, lighted tube with a camera.

- **Biologic Therapy:** Medications derived from living organisms that target specific molecules involved in inflammation and immune response.

- **Fecal Microbiota Transplantation (FMT):** A procedure that involves transferring fecal matter from a healthy donor to the gastrointestinal tract of a recipient to restore microbial balance.

- **Mesenchymal Stem Cells (MSCs):** Multipotent cells found in various tissues, including bone marrow and adipose tissue, with the potential to differentiate into different cell types and modulate immune responses.

- **Patient-Centered Outcomes Research:** Research that focuses on identifying and prioritizing outcomes that matter most to patients, such as symptom control, quality of life, and treatment satisfaction.

3. Further Reading

1. **Books:**

   - "Living with Crohn's & Colitis: A Comprehensive Naturopathic Guide for Complete Digestive Wellness" by Dede Cummings and Jessica Black

   - "Crohn's and Colitis: Understanding and Managing IBD" by Hillary Steinhart

   - "The First Year: Crohn's Disease and Ulcerative Colitis: An Essential Guide for the Newly Diagnosed" by Jill Sklar and M.D. Cheifetz

2. **Scientific Journals:**

   - "Inflammatory Bowel Diseases" (Journal)

   - "Gastroenterology" (Journal)

   - "Clinical Gastroenterology and Hepatology" (Journal)

3. **Online Articles:**

   - "Ulcerative Colitis Overview" - Mayo Clinic: mayoclinic.org/diseases-conditions/ulcerative-colitis

   - "Ulcerative Colitis" - Centres for Disease Control and Prevention (CDC): cdc.gov/ibd/what-is-IBD/ulcerative-colitis

Conclusion

The appendices provide valuable resources, a glossary of key terms, and further reading materials for individuals interested in learning more about ulcerative colitis (UC). Whether seeking support, educational materials, or scientific literature, these resources offer valuable information and insights to empower individuals with UC and enhance their understanding of this complex condition.